Vegetarian Diet Made Easy 2021

Easy, Tasty and Low Cost Recipes for Every Meal to Lose Weight, Burn Fat and Transform Your Body

Grace Young

© **Copyright 2021 - Grace Young - All rights reserved.**

The content contained within this book may not be reproduced, duplicated or transmitted without direct written permission from the author or the publisher.

Under no circumstances will any blame or legal responsibility be held against the publisher, or author, for any damages, reparation, or monetary loss due to the information contained within this book. Either directly or indirectly.

Legal Notice:

This book is copyright protected. This book is only for personal use. You cannot amend, distribute, sell, use, quote or paraphrase any part, or the content within this book, without the consent of the author or publisher.

Disclaimer Notice:

Please note the information contained within this document is for educational and entertainment purposes only. All effort has been executed to present accurate, up to date, and reliable, complete information. No warranties of any kind are declared or implied. Readers acknowledge that the author is not engaging in the rendering of legal, financial, medical or professional advice. The content within this book has been derived from various sources. Please consult a licensed professional before attempting any techniques outlined in this book.

By reading this document, the reader agrees that under no circumstances is the author responsible for any losses, direct or indirect, which are incurred as a result of the use of information contained within this document, including, but not limited to, — errors, omissions, or inaccuracies

Table of Content

BREAKFASTS 9
- ORANGE DREAM CREAMSICLE 11
- STRAWBERRY LIMEADE 12
- PEANUT BUTTER AND JELLY SMOOTHIE 13
- BANANA BREAD BREAKFAST MUFFINS 14
- STRACCIATELLA MUFFINS 16
- CARDAMOM PERSIMMON SCONES WITH MAPLE-PERSIMMON CREAM 17
- QUINOA APPLESAUCE MUFFINS 19
- PUMPKIN PANCAKES 21
- GREEN BREAKFAST SMOOTHIE 23

ENTRÉES 25
- OVEN BAKED SESAME FRIES 26
- PUMPKIN ORANGE SPICE HUMMUS 27

SOUPS, SALADS, AND SIDES 29
- NOURISHING WHOLE-GRAIN PORRIDGE 30
- PUNGENT MUSHROOM BARLEY RISOTTO 31
- ARUGULA LENTIL SALAD 33
- RED CABBAGE SALAD WITH CURRIED SEITAN 35

LUNCH RECIPES 37
- AVOCADO AND HUMMUS SANDWICH 39
- CHICKPEA SPINACH SALAD 40
- VEGGIE FRITTERS 41
- PIZZA BITES 43
- SPINACH AND BROCCOLI SOUP 45
- COCONUT ZUCCHINI CREAM 46
- ZUCCHINI AND CAULIFLOWER SOUP 48

DINNER RECIPES 50
- 50
- SMOKED TEMPEH WITH BROCCOLI FRITTERS 51
- CHEESY POTATO CASSEROLE 53
- SPICY CHEESY TOFU BALLS 54
- MANGO STICKY RICE 56
- SPICY GRILLED TOFU STEAK 57

Piquillo Salsa Verde Steak	59

SMOOTHIES, SNACKS AND DESSERTS 61

Berry & Cauliflower Smoothie	62
Green Mango Smoothie	63
Chia Seed Smoothie	64
Mango Smoothie	65
Beans with Sesame Hummus	66
Hazelnut & Maple Chia Crunch	67
Honey Peanut Butter	68
Mediterranean Marinated Olives	69
Nut Butter & Dates Granola	70
Oven-baked Caramelize Plantains	71
Powerful Peas & Lentils Dip	72
Avocado Hummus	73
Plant Based Crispy Falafel	74
Waffles With Almond Flour	76
Avocado And Tempeh Bacon Wraps	77
Kale Chips	78
Apple Cinnamon Crisps	79

FLAVOUR BOOSTERS AND SOUCE RECIPES 80

Southwestern Oregano Thyme Rub	80
Tangy Pepper & Thyme Rub	82
Vegan Smokey Maple BBQ Sauce	83
Vegan Bean Pesto	84

MEAL PLANS 85

Meal Plan 1	85
Meal Plan 2	90
Meal Plan 3	95
Meal plan 4	99

Breakfasts

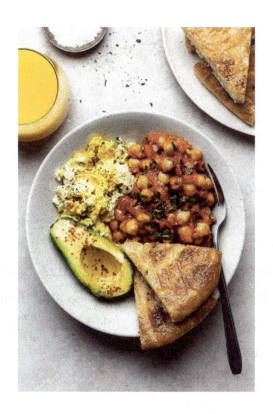

Green Ginger Smoothie

Preparation time: 5 minutes

Cooking time: 5 minutes

Servings: 2

Ingredients:

1 banana

½ apple sliced

1 orange sliced and peeled

1 lemon juice

2 big spinach

1 tbsp. fresh ginger

½ cup almond milk

For the dressing: chia seeds, apple, raspberries

Directions:

Take a blender. Peel off and slice all fruits. Add banana, apple, orange, lime juice, ginger and spinach and blend them well until they turn smooth. Now add almond milk and pulse again for a few seconds. Pour the smoothie into glasses and serve. You can add chia seeds, apple or raspberries for a smoothie bowl. Store it up to 8-10 hours in the refrigerator.

Nutrition: Calories 330 Carbohydrates 62 g Fats 6 g Protein 10 g

Orange Dream Creamsicle

Preparation time: 5 minutes

Cooking time: 5 minutes

Servings: 2

Ingredients:

1 orange, peeled

¼ cup vegan yogurt

2 tbsp. orange juice

¼ tsp vanilla extract

4 ice cubes

Directions:

In a blender, add orange, orange juice, vegan yogurt, vanilla extract and ice cubes. Blend all the ingredients well until smooth and well combined. Pour it into smoothie glasses and serve.

Nutrition: Calories 120 Carbohydrates 62 g Fats 6 g Protein 10g

Strawberry Limeade

Preparation time: 5 minutes

Cooking time: 5 minutes

Servings: 6

Ingredients:

2 cup strawberries

1 cup sugar or as per taste

7 cups of water

2 cup lemon juice

Sliced berries for garnish

Directions:

Take a small bowl, add sugar and water and put in microwave until dissolved. Now take a blender and add strawberries and a cup of water and blend well. Combine the strawberries puree with the sugar dissolve water and mix. Pour lime juice and water if required. Stir well and chill before serving. You can add berries on the top as garnishing.

Nutrition: Calories: 144, carbohydrates: 37g, sugar: 35g

Peanut Butter and Jelly Smoothie

Preparation time: 5 minutes

Cooking time: 5 minutes

Servings: 2

Ingredients:

1 cup frozen raspberries

1 cup frozen strawberries

1 serving collagen peptides

1 tbsp. peanut butter

¾ cup almond milk

Directions:

Take a blender. Add in raspberries, strawberries, peanut butter, collagen peptide and almond milk. Blend all ingredients until well combined. Add almond milk as per the required consistency. Pour into smoothie serving glasses and top up with the peanut butter or anything of your choice for dressing.

Nutrition: Calories: 251, fat: 11.1g, carbohydrates: 27.5g, proteins: 15.7g

Banana Bread Breakfast Muffins

Preparation time: 40 m

Cooking time: 20 m

Ingredients:

1/2 cup plus 2 tbs of whole oats

1/2 cup oats (processed into flour)

1/2 teaspoon baking powder

2 tablespoon vegan chocolate chips

1/4 teaspoon cinnamon

1/2 cup of a mashed ripe banana (mash the banana and then measure it)

2 tablespoons pure maple syrup

1/2 teaspoon vanilla extract

Directions:

Preheat the cooker to 360 ° F and spray a muffin pan (3-4 holes) with a non-stick spray.

Add 1/2 cup oatmeal in a food processor and beat until it breaks and forms a thick consistency of flour.

In a large container, add all the dry ingredients except the chocolate chips and mix.

Crush and mash the uneven ripe banana, add the banana and the rest of the wet ingredients to the container with the dry ingredients and mix well.

Mix the chocolate chips. Put in 3-4 muffin holes and bake for 12 minutes.

Let cool 10 mins and serve immediately or store in an airtight container for 1-2 days.

Nutrition: Per serving: Carbohydrates: 59g Calories: 347 Fat: 6g Sodium: 2 mg Proteins: 15g Sugar: 1g

Stracciatella Muffins

Preparation time: 30 m

Cooking time: 15 m

Ingredients:

1 tablespoon vinegar

1 cup of soy milk

8 1/2-ounces flour

3/4-ounce grams brown sugar

3 1/2-ounces white sugar

2 packs of vanilla sugar

1/2 teaspoon salt

1 package baking soda

5-ounces vegan chocolate chip or finely grated chocolate (bittersweet)

2 tablespoons oil

Directions:

Preheat the oven to 355 ° F.

Mix the soy milk together with the vinegar and set aside.

In a large bowl, pour the flour, sugar, vanilla sugar, baking powder, and salt. Add the soybean oil and milk and mix until you get a smooth paste (with a spoon, not the blender). Carefully fold the chocolate chips. Divide into 12 prepared muffin shapes and bake for 18 to 20 minutes until a toothpick comes out without sticky dough residue.

Nutrition: Per serving: Carbohydrates: 26 g Calories: 132 Fat: 7g Sodium: 17 mg Proteins: 2 g Sugar: 15 g

Cardamom Persimmon Scones With Maple-Persimmon Cream

Preparation time: 45 m

Cooking time: 30 m

Ingredients:

For the Dry Ingredients:

2 teaspoons baking powder

1 tablespoon coconut sugar

1 teaspoon cardamom

1/2 teaspoon salt

1/2 teaspoon cinnamon

3 tablespoons softened coconut oil

For the Wet Ingredients:

1/2 cup almond milk

1 teaspoon vanilla extract

1 cup plain vegan yogurt

1 teaspoon apple cider vinegar (if you use vegan yogurt)

1 cup ripe Fuyu persimmons chopped

For the Maple Cream:

2 tablespoons shredded coconut

1/2 cup chopped persimmons

3/4 cup non-dairy milk

1/4 teaspoon cinnamon

1 tablespoon maple syrup

1/4 teaspoon salt

Directions:

For Scones:

Preheat the cooker to 400 ° F. Line a baking sheet with parchment paper or leave it bare.

Combine flour, sugar, spices, baking soda, and salt in a large bowl.

Using a fork or pasta cutter, cut the coconut oil into the mixture.

Combine yogurt, almond milk, apple cider vinegar, and vanilla in a small bowl. Add the dey ingredients to the wet ingredients and stir with a wooden spoon until the mixture is well combined. Be careful not to mix too much.

Gently fold the chopped persimmons with the wooden spoon. Flour on a flat surface like a board or a counter. Make the dough in a circle about 1.2 cm high. Cut into 8 slices and separate. Carefully transfer the slices to the prepared baking sheet. Bake at 400 ° F for 18 to 20 minutes. Let cool slightly before serving. For the cream: Combine all the constituents in a blender or food processor.

Serve with hot scones or refrigerate for up to 3 days.

Nutrition: Per serving: Carbohydrates: 45g Calories: 264 Fat: 7g Sodium: 46 mg Proteins: 6g Sugar: 15g

Quinoa Applesauce Muffins

Preparation time: 10 minutes

Cooking time: 15 minutes

Servings: 5

Ingredients

2 tablespoons coconut oil or margarine, melted, plus more for coating the muffin tin

¼ Cup ground flaxseed

½ Cup water

2 cups unsweetened applesauce

½ Cup brown sugar

1 teaspoon apple cider vinegar

2½ cups whole-grain flour

1½ cups cooked quinoa

2 teaspoons baking soda

Pinch salt

½ Cup dried cranberries or raisins

Directions

Preheat the oven to 400°f.

Coat a muffin tin with coconut oil, line with paper muffin cups, or use a nonstick tin. In a large bowl, stir together the flaxseed and water. Add the applesauce, sugar, coconut oil, and vinegar. Stir to combine. Add the flour, quinoa, baking soda, and salt, stirring until just combined. Gently fold in the cranberries without stirring too much. Scoop the muffin mixture into the prepared tin, about ⅓ cup for each muffin.

Bake for 15 to 20 minutes, until slightly browned on top and springy to the touch. Let cool for about 10 minutes. Run a dinner knife around the inside of each cup to loosen, then tilt the muffins on their sides in the muffin wells so air gets underneath. These keep in an airtight container in the refrigerator for up to 1 week or in the freezer indefinitely.

Per serving (1 muffin): calories: 387; protein: 7g; total fat: 5g; saturated fat: 2g; carbohydrates: 57g; fiber: 8g

Pumpkin Pancakes

Preparation time: 15 minutes

Cooking time: 15 minutes

Servings: 4

Ingredients

2 cups unsweetened almond milk

1 teaspoon apple cider vinegar

2½ cups whole-wheat flour

2 tablespoons baking powder

½ Teaspoon baking soda

1 teaspoon sea salt

1 teaspoon pumpkin pie spice or ½ teaspoon ground -cinnamon plus ¼ teaspoon grated -nutmeg plus ¼ teaspoon ground allspice

½ Cup canned pumpkin purée

1 cup water

1 tablespoon coconut oil

Directions

In a small bowl, combine the almond milk and apple cider vinegar. Set aside.

In a bowl, whisk together the flour, baking powder, baking soda, salt, and pumpkin pie spice. In bowl, combine the almond milk mixture, pumpkin purée, and water, whisking to mix well. Mix the wet Ingredients to the dry Ingredients and fold together until the dry -Ingredients are just moistened.

In a nonstick pan or griddle over medium-high heat, melt the coconut oil and swirl to coat. Pour the batter into the pan ¼ cup at a time and cook until the pancakes are browned, about 5 minutes per side. Serve immediately.

Green Breakfast Smoothie

Preparation time: 10 minutes

Cooking time: 0 minutes

Servings: 2

Ingredients

½ Banana, sliced

2 cups spinach or other greens, such as kale

1 cup sliced berries of your choosing, fresh or frozen

1 orange, peeled and cut into segments

1 cup unsweetened nondairy milk

1 cup ice

Directions

In a blender, combine all the Ingredients.

Starting with the blender on low speed, begin blending the smoothie, gradually increasing blender speed until smooth. Serve immediately.

Entrées

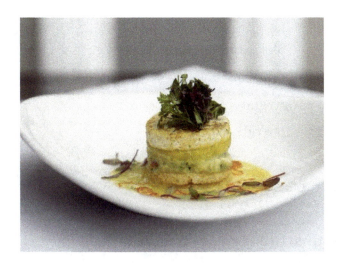

Oven Baked Sesame Fries

Preparation time: 30 minutes

Cooking time: 30 minutes

Servings: 4

Ingredients:

1 pound Yukon Gold potatoes, skins on and cut into wedges

2 tablespoons sesame seeds

1 tablespoon potato starch

1 tablespoon sesame oil

Salt to taste

Black pepper to taste

Directions:

Preheat the oven to 425 degrees, Fahrenheit and cover a baking sheet or two with parchment paper.

Cut the potatoes and place in a large bowl.

Add the sesame seeds, potato starch, sesame oil, salt and pepper.

Toss with your hands and make sure all the wedges are coated. Add more sesame seeds or oil if needed.

Spread the potato wedges on the baking sheets with some room between each wedge.

Bake for 15 minutes, flip the wedges over and then return them to the oven for 10 to 15 more minutes, until they look golden and crispy.

Pumpkin Orange Spice Hummus

Preparation 30 minutes Cooking 30 minutes Servings: 3

Ingredients:

1 cup canned, unsweetened pumpkin puree

1 16-ounce can garbanzo beans, rinsed and drained

1 tablespoon apple cider vinegar

1 tablespoon maple syrup

¼ cup tahini

1 tablespoon fresh orange juice

½ teaspoon orange zest and additional zest for garnish

⅛ teaspoon ground cinnamon

⅛ teaspoon ground ginger

⅛ teaspoon ground nutmeg

¼ teaspoon salt

Directions: Pour the pumpkin puree and garbanzo beans into a food processor and pulse to break up. Add the vinegar, syrup, tahini, orange juice and orange zest pulse a few times. Add the cinnamon, ginger, nutmeg and salt and process until smooth and creamy. Serve in a bowl sprinkled with more orange zest with wheat crackers alongside.

Soups, Salads, and Sides

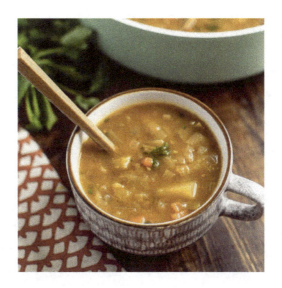

Nourishing Whole-Grain Porridge

Preparation time: 2 hours and 10 minutes

Cooking time: 2 hours

Servings: 4

Ingredients:

3/4 cup of steel-cut oats, rinsed and soaked overnight

3/4 cup of whole barley, rinsed and soaked overnight

1/2 cup of cornmeal

1 teaspoon of salt

3 tablespoons of brown sugar

1 cinnamon stick, about 3 inches long

1 teaspoon of vanilla extract, unsweetened

4 1/2 cups of water

Directions:

Using a 6-quarts slow cooker, place all the ingredients and stir properly.

Cover it with the lid, plug in the slow cooker and let it cook for 2 hours or until grains get soft, while stirring halfway through. Serve the porridge with fruits.

Nutrition: Calories: 129 Cal, Carbohydrates:22g, Protein:5g, Fats:2g, Fiber:4g.

Pungent Mushroom Barley Risotto

Preparation time: 3 hours and 30 minutes

Cooking time: 3 hours and 9 minutes

Servings: 4

Ingredients:

1 1/2 cups of hulled barley, rinsed and soaked overnight

8 ounces of carrots, peeled and chopped

1 pound of mushrooms, sliced

1 large white onion, peeled and chopped

3/4 teaspoon of salt

1/2 teaspoon of ground black pepper

4 sprigs thyme

1/4 cup of chopped parsley

2/3 cup of grated vegan Parmesan cheese

1 tablespoon of apple cider vinegar

2 tablespoons of olive oil

1 1/2 cups of vegetable broth

Directions:

Place a large non-stick skillet pan over a medium-high heat, add the oil and let it heat until it gets hot.

Add the onion along with 1/4 teaspoon of each the salt and black pepper.

Cook it for 5 minutes or until it turns golden brown.

Then add the mushrooms and continue cooking for 2 minutes.

Add the barley, thyme and cook for another 2 minutes.

Transfer this mixture to a 6-quarts slow cooker and add the carrots, 1/4 teaspoon of salt, and the vegetable broth.

Stir properly and cover it with the lid.

Plug in the slow cooker, let it cook for 3 hours at the high heat setting or until the grains absorb all the cooking liquid and the vegetables get soft.

Remove the thyme sprigs, pour in the remaining ingredients except for parsley and stir properly.

Pour in the warm water and stir properly until the risotto reaches your desired state.

Add the seasoning, then garnish it with parsley and serve.

Nutrition: Calories:321 Cal, Carbohydrates:48g, Protein:12g, Fats:10g, Fiber:11g.

Arugula Lentil Salad

Preparation time: 5 mins.

Cooking time: 5 mins.

Ingredient: ¾ cups cashews (¾ cups = 100 g)
- 1 onion
- 3 tbsp olive oil
- 1 chilli / jalapeño
- 5-6 sun-dried tomatoes in oil
- 3 slices bread (whole wheat)
- 1 cup brown lentils, cooked (1 cup = 1 / 15oz / 400 g)
- 1 handful arugula/rocket (1 handful = 100 g)
- 1-2 tbsp balsamic vinegar
- salt and pepper to taste.

Directions:

Roast the cashews on a low heat for about three minutes in a pan to maximize aroma. Then throw them into the salad bowl. Dice up and fry the onion in one third of the olive oil for about 3 minutes on a low heat. Meanwhile chop the chilli/jalapeño and dried tomatoes. Add them to the pan and fry for another 1-2 minutes. Cut the bread into big croutons. Move the onion mix into a big bowl. Now add the rest of the oil to the pan and fry the chopped-up bread until crunchy. Season with salt and pepper. Wash the arugula and add it to the bowl. Put the lentils in too, and mix them all around. Season with salt, pepper and balsamic vinegar. Serve with the croutons. Super tasty!

Red Cabbage Salad With Curried Seitan

Preparation 10 mins Cooking 10 mins

Ingredient:

    1 Tbs. olive oil

    1 8-oz. pkg. seitan, cut into bite-size strips

    3 cloves garlic, minced (1 Tbs.)

    ¾ tsp. mild curry powder

    6 cups shredded red cabbage (½ small head)

    1 small cucumber, sliced into thin half-moons (¾ cup)

    3 green onions, thinly sliced (½ cup)

    ⅓ cup prepared mango chutney

    ⅓ cup creamy natural peanut butter.

Directions: To make Dressing: Blend chutney, peanut butter, and 1/3 cup water in blender until smooth. Set aside. To make Salad: Heat 2 tsp. oil in large skillet over medium heat. Add seitan, and season with salt, if desired. Sauté 5 to 7 minutes, or until browned. Add garlic and remaining 1 tsp. oil, and sauté 30 seconds. Sprinkle with curry powder, and sauté 2 minutes more. Remove from heat, and keep warm. Toss cabbage and cucumber with Dressing in large bowl. Top with warm seitan and green onions.

Lunch Recipes

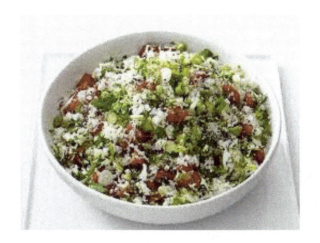

Cauliflower Steaks

Preparation Time: 10 minutes Cooking Time: 30 minutes

Serving: 3

Ingredients:

2 medium heads of cauliflower

1 teaspoon garlic powder

1/2 teaspoon ground black pepper

1 teaspoon salt

1 teaspoon coriander

1 teaspoon paprika

2 tablespoons olive oil

For Serving:

1 cup (236 grams) hummus

Directions:

Switch on the oven, set it to 425° F and let it preheat. Cut each cauliflower head into three slices, brush them with oil on both sides and sprinkle with garlic powder, black pepper, salt, coriander, and paprika. Take a large baking sheet, line it with aluminum foil, arrange cauliflower steaks on it and then bake for 30 minutes until tender and golden brown on both sides. Serve straight away.

Nutrition: 149 Cal; 9 g Fat; 1 g Saturated Fat; 14 g Carbs; 7 g Fiber; 5 g Protein; 3 g Sugar;

Avocado And Hummus Sandwich

Preparation Time: 5 minutes

Cooking Time: 0 minutes

Serving: 1

Ingredients:

2 slices of whole-wheat bread sliced

4 slices of tomato

1 lettuce leaf

1/2 avocado, sliced

2 tablespoons cilantro leaves

2 teaspoons hot sauce

3 tablespoon hummus

Directions:

Take a slice of bread, spread hummus on its one side, then top with avocado slices and drizzle with hot sauce.

Scatter tomato slice on top of avocado slices, then top with lettuce and cilantro and cover with the other slice of bread. Serve straight away.

Nutrition: 302 Cal; 5.7 g Fat; 1.1 g Saturated Fat; 49.8 g Carbs; 12 g Fiber; 12.8 g Protein; 7.8 g Sugar;

Chickpea Spinach Salad

Preparation Time: 10 minutes Cooking Time: 0 minutes

Serving: 2

Ingredients:

12 ounces (340 grams) cooked chickpeas

1/4 cup (59 grams) raisins

1 cup (236 grams) spinach

1/2 teaspoon red chili flakes

1/8 teaspoon salt

1 teaspoon cumin

3 teaspoons agave syrup

1/2 tablespoon lemon juice

4 tablespoons olive oil

3 ½ ounces (99 grams) vegan parmesan cheese

Directions:

Take a large salad bowl, add chickpeas and spinach in it, then add cheese and toss until mixed. Prepare the dressing: take a small bowl, add raisins in it along with salt, pepper, cumin, lemon juice, agave syrup and oil and whisk until combined. Drizzle the dressing over salad, toss until well coated, and serve.

Nutrition: 658 Cal; 40 g Fat; 11 g Saturated Fat; 52 g Carbs; 9.7 g Fiber; 23 g Protein; 15.2 g Sugar;

Veggie Fritters

Preparation Time: 35 Minutes

Cooking Time: 20 Minutes

Servings: 4

Ingredients:

Flour (2 C.)

Cabbage (4 C., Cut)

Carrots (2 C., Sliced)

Shallots (3)

Water (1.25 C.)

Garlic Cloves (3)

Olive Oil (2 T.)

Salt (to Taste)

Powdered Mushroom Stock (15 t.)

Pepper (to Taste)

Directions:

You will want to begin this recipe by crushing the pepper, salt, mushroom powder, garlic, and shallots together. By the end, you should have created a paste.

In another bowl, go ahead and mix together the paste, water, carrot slices, cabbage., and the flour together. From this, you will be creating a thick, chunky batter.

Now that your batter is made, you'll want to begin to heat a pan over medium heat and then place the oil in once warm. As the oil begins to sizzle, create 1-inch patties with your batter and lay them in the pan like pancakes. After frying the patty for five minutes on one side, flip it over and cook the other side until both sides reach a nice golden color.

Once you are done cooking, pat the fritter down with a paper towel to remove excess oil, and then you can enjoy!

Nutrition: Calories: 330 Proteins: 10g Carbs: 60g Fats: 6g

Pizza Bites

Preparation Time: 1 Hour

Cooking Time: 30 Minutes

Servings: 4

Ingredients:

Olive Oil (1 t.)

Dried Oregano (1 t.)

Lemon Juice (1 t.)

Dried Basil (1 t.)

Tomato Sauce (1 C.)

Cauliflower (1 Head)

Salt (to Taste)

Nutritional Yeast (to Taste)

Garlic Cloves (2, Minced)

Directions:

Begin by prepping the oven to 300 and line a pan with parchment paper. When this is set, take a mixing bowl and combine the olive oil, oregano, basil, salt, tomato sauce, and the basil together. In a second bowl, you will want to place your nutritional yeast.

When you are ready, gently dip the cauliflower pieces into the tomato sauce and then roll in the nutritional yeast. You will want to place these on the baking sheet and continue until all of the cauliflower is covered.

Once the cauliflower is set, place it into the oven for about an hour or until the edges are crispy. Once they are cooked to your liking, remove from the oven and enjoy with some extra sauce for dipping!

Nutrition: Calories: 110 Proteins: 5g Carbs: 17g Fats: 3g

Spinach and Broccoli Soup

Preparation time: 10 minutes

Cooking time: 20 minutes

Servings: 4

Ingredients:

3 shallots, chopped

1 tablespoon olive oil

2 garlic cloves, minced

½ pound broccoli florets

½ pound baby spinach

Salt and black pepper to the taste

4 cups veggie stock

1 teaspoon turmeric powder

1 tablespoon lime juice

Directions:

Heat up a pot with the oil over medium high heat, add the shallots and the garlic and sauté for 5 minutes.

Add the broccoli, spinach and the other ingredients, toss, bring to a simmer and cook over medium heat for 15 minutes.

Ladle into soup bowls and serve.

Nutrition: calories 150, fat 3, fiber 1, carbs 3, protein 7

Coconut zucchini cream

Preparation time: 10 minutes

Cooking time: 25 minutes

Servings: 4

Ingredients:

1 pound zucchinis, roughly chopped

2 tablespoons avocado oil

4 scallions, chopped

Salt and black pepper to the taste

6 cups veggie stock

1 teaspoon basil, dried

1 teaspoon cumin, ground

3 garlic cloves, minced

¾ cup coconut cream

1 tablespoon dill, chopped

Directions:

Heat up a pot with the oil over medium high heat, add the scallions and the garlic and sauté for 5 minutes.

Add the rest of the ingredients, stir, bring to a simmer and cook over medium heat for 20 minutes more.

Blend the soup using an immersion blender, ladle into bowls and serve.

Nutrition: calories 160, fat 4, fiber 2, carbs 4, protein 8

Zucchini and Cauliflower Soup

Preparation time: 10 minutes

Cooking time: 25 minutes

Servings: 4

Ingredients:

4 scallions, chopped

1 teaspoon ginger, grated

2 tablespoons olive oil

1 pound zucchinis, sliced

2 cups cauliflower florets

Salt and black pepper to the taste

6 cups veggie stock

1 garlic clove, minced

1 tablespoon lemon juice

1 cup coconut cream

Directions:

Heat up a pot with the oil over medium heat, add the scallions, ginger and the garlic and sauté for 5 minutes.

Add the rest of the ingredients, bring to a simmer and cook over medium heat for 20 minutes.

Blend everything using an immersion blender, ladle into soup bowls and serve.

Nutrition: calories 154, fat 12, fiber 3, carbs 5, protein 4

Dinner Recipes

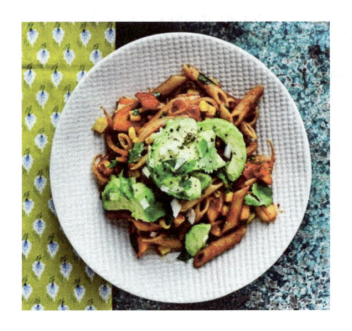

Smoked Tempeh with Broccoli Fritters

Preparation Time: 25 minutes

Cooking Time: 20 minutes

Servings: 4

Ingredients:

For the flax egg:

4 tbsp flax seed powder + 12 tbsp water

For the grilled tempeh:

3 tbsp olive oil

1 tbsp soy sauce

3 tbsp fresh lime juice

1 tbsp grated ginger

Salt and cayenne pepper to taste

10 oz. tempeh slices

For the broccoli fritters:

2 cups of rice broccoli

8 oz. tofu cheese

3 tbsp plain flour

½ tsp onion powder

1 tsp salt

¼ tsp freshly ground black pepper

4¼ oz. vegan butter

For serving:

½ cup mixed salad greens

1 cup vegan mayonnaise

½ lemon, juiced

Directions:

For the smoked tempeh:

In a bowl, mix the flax seed powder with water and set aside to soak for 5 minutes.

In another bowl, combine the olive oil, soy sauce, lime juice, grated ginger, salt, and cayenne pepper. Brush the tempeh slices with the mixture.

Heat a grill pan over medium heat and grill the tempeh on both sides until nicely smoked and golden brown, 8 minutes. Transfer to a plate and set aside in a warmer for serving.

In a medium bowl, combine the broccoli rice, tofu cheese, flour, onion, salt, and black pepper. Mix in the flax egg until well combine and form 1-inch thick patties out of the mixture. Melt the vegan butter in a medium skillet over medium heat and fry the patties on both sides until golden brown, 8 minutes. Remove the fritters onto a plate and set aside.

In a small bowl, mix the vegan mayonnaise with the lemon juice.

Divide the smoked tempeh and broccoli fritters onto serving plates, add the salad greens, and serve with the vegan mayonnaise sauce.

Cheesy Potato Casserole

Preparation Time: 30 minutes

Cooking Time: 20 minutes

Servings: 4

Ingredients:

2 oz. vegan butter

½ cup celery stalks, finely chopped

1 white onion, finely chopped

1 green bell pepper, seeded and finely chopped

Salt and black pepper to taste

2 cups peeled and chopped potatoes

1 cup vegan mayonnaise

4 oz. freshly shredded vegan Parmesan cheese

1 tsp red chili flakes

Directions:

Preheat the oven to 400 F and grease a baking dish with cooking spray. Season the celery, onion, and bell pepper with salt and black pepper. In a bowl, mix the potatoes, vegan mayonnaise, Parmesan cheese, and red chili flakes. Pour the mixture into the baking dish, add the season vegetables, and mix well. Bake in the oven until golden brown, about 20 minutes.

Remove the baked potato and serve warm with baby spinach.

Spicy Cheesy Tofu Balls

Preparation Time: 30 minutes

Cooking Time: 15 minutes

Servings: 4

Ingredients:

1/3 cup vegan mayonnaise

1/4 cup pickled jalapenos

1 pinch cayenne pepper

4 oz. grated vegan cheddar cheese

1 tsp paprika powder

1 tbsp mustard powder

1 tbsp flax seed powder + 3 tbsp water

2 1/2 cup crumbled tofu

Salt and black pepper to taste

2 tbsp vegan butter, for frying

Directions:

For the spicy cheese:

In a bowl, mix all the ingredients for the spicy vegan cheese until well combined. Set aside.

In another medium bowl, combine the flax seed powder with water and allow soaking for 5 minutes.

Add the flax egg to the cheese mixture, the crumbled tofu, salt, and black pepper, and combine well. Use your hands to form large meatballs out of the mix.

Melt the vegan butter in a large skillet over medium heat and fry the tofu balls until cooked and golden brown on all sides, 10 minutes.

Serve the tofu balls with your favorite mashes or in burgers.

Mango Sticky Rice

Preparation Time: 35 Minutes

Cooking Time: 30 Minutes

Servings: 3

Calories: 571

Protein: 6 Grams

Fat: 29.6 Grams

Carbs: 77.6 Grams

Ingredients:

½ Cup Sugar

1 Mango, Sliced

14 Ounces Coconut Milk, Canned

½ Cup Basmati Rice

Directions:

Cook your rice per package instructions, and add half of your sugar. When cooking your rice, substitute half of your water for half of your coconut milk.

Boil your remaining coconut milk in a saucepan with your remaining sugar.

Boil on high heat until it's thick, and then add in your mango slices.

Interesting Facts: Mangos contain 50% of the daily Vitamin C you should consume which aid in bone and immune health.

Spicy Grilled Tofu Steak

Preparation Time: 30 min.

Cooking Time: 20 min.

Servings: 4

Ingredients:

1 tbsp. of the following:

chopped scallion

chopped cilantro

soy sauce

hoisin sauce

2 tbsp. oil

¼ t. of the following:

salt

garlic powder

red chili pepper powder

ground Sichuan peppercorn powder

½ t. cumin

1 pound firm tofu

Directions:

Place the tofu on a plate and drain the excess liquid for about 10 minutes.

Slice drained tofu into ¾ thick stakes.

Stir the cumin, Sichuan peppercorn, chili powder, garlic powder, and salt in a mixing bowl until well-incorporated.

In another little bowl, combine soy sauce, hoisin, and 1 teaspoon of oil.

Heat a skillet to medium temperature with oil, then carefully place the tofu in the skillet.

Sprinkle the spices over the tofu, distributing equally across all steaks. Cook for 3-5 minutes, flip, and put spice on the other side. Cook for an additional 3 minutes.

Brush with sauce and plate.

Sprinkle some scallion and cilantro and enjoy.

Nutrition: Calories: 155 | Carbohydrates: 7.6 g | Proteins: 9.9 g | Fats: 11.8g

Piquillo Salsa Verde Steak

Preparation Time: 30 min.

Cooking Time: 25 min.

Yields: 8 Servings

Ingredients:

4 – ½ inch thick slices of ciabatta

18 oz. firm tofu, drained

5 tbsp. olive oil, extra virgin

Pinch of cayenne

½ t. cumin, ground

1 ½ tbsp. sherry vinegar

1 shallot, diced

8 piquillo peppers (can be from a jar) – drained and cut to ½ inch strips

3 tbsp. of the following:

parsley, finely chopped

capers, drained and chopped

Directions:

Place the tofu on a plate to drain the excess liquid, and then slice into 8 rectangle pieces.

You can either prepare your grill or use a grill pan. If using a grill pan, preheat the grill pan.

Mix 3 tablespoons of olive oil, cayenne, cumin, vinegar, shallot, parsley, capers, and piquillo peppers in a medium bowl to make our salsa verde. Season to preference with salt and pepper.

Using a paper towel, dry the tofu slices.

Brush olive oil on each side, seasoning with salt and pepper lightly.

Place the bread on the grill and toast for about 2 minutes using medium-high heat.

Next, grill the tofu, cooking each side for about 3 minutes or until the tofu is heated through.

Place the toasted bread on the plate then the tofu on top of the bread.

Gently spoon out the salsa verde over the tofu and serve.

Nutrition: Calories: 427 | Carbohydrates: 67.5 g | Proteins: 14.2 g | Fats: 14.6 g

Smoothies, Snacks and Desserts

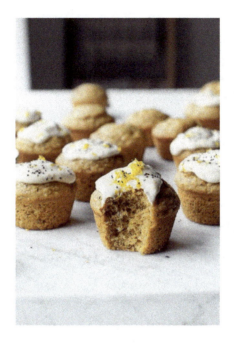

Berry & Cauliflower Smoothie

Preparation Time: 10 Minutes

Cooking Time: 0 minutes

Serves: 2

Calories: 149

Protein: 3 Grams

Fat: 3 Grams

Carbs: 29 Grams

Ingredients:

1 Cup Riced Cauliflower, Frozen

1 Cup Banana, Sliced & Frozen

½ Cup Mixed Berries, Frozen

2 Cups Almond Milk, Unsweetened

2 Teaspoons Maple syrup, Pure & Optional

Directions:

Blend until mixed well.

Green Mango Smoothie

Preparation Time: 5 Minutes

Cooking Time: 0 minutes

Serves: 1

Calories: 417

Protein: 7.2 Grams

Fat: 2.8 Grams

Carbs: 102.8 Grams

Ingredients:

2 Cups Spinach

1-2 Cups Coconut Water

2 Mangos, Ripe, Peeled & Diced

Directions:

Blend everything together until smooth.

Chia Seed Smoothie

Preparation Time: 5 Minutes

Cooking Time: 0 minutes

Serves: 3

Calories: 477

Protein: 8 Grams

Fat: 29 Grams

Carbs: 57 Grams

Ingredients:

¼ Teaspoon Cinnamon

1 Tablespoon Ginger, Fresh & Grated

Pinch Cardamom

1 Tablespoon Chia Seeds

2 Medjool Dates, Pitted

1 Cup Alfalfa Sprouts

1 Cup Water

1 Banana

½ Cup Coconut Milk, Unsweetened

Directions:

Blend everything together until smooth.

Mango Smoothie

Preparation Time: 5 Minutes

Cooking Time: 0 minutes

Serves: 3

Calories: 376

Protein: 5 Grams

Fat: 2 Grams

Carbs: 95 Grams

Ingredients:

1 Carrot, Peeled & Chopped

1 Cup Strawberries

1 Cup Water

1 Cup Peaches, Chopped

1 Banana, Frozen & sliced

1 Cup Mango, Chopped

Directions:

Blend everything together until smooth.

Beans with Sesame Hummus

Preparation time: 10 minutes

Cooking time: 0 minutes

Servings: 6

Ingredients

4 Tbsp sesame oil

2 cloves garlic finely sliced

1 can (15 oz) cannellini beans, drained

4 Tbsp sesame paste

2 Tbsp lemon juice freshly squeezed

1/4 tsp red pepper flakes

2 Tbsp fresh basil finely chopped

2 Tbsp fresh parsley finely chopped

Sea salt to taste

Directions:

Place all ingredients in your food processor.

Process until all ingredients are combined well and smooth.

Transfer mixture into a bowl and refrigerate until servings.

Hazelnut & Maple Chia Crunch

Preparation Time: 30 Minutes

Cooking Time: 5 Minutes

Servings: 2

Ingredients:

Chia Seeds (.25 C.)

Olive Oil (1 t.)

Maple Syrup (.50 C.)

Hazelnuts (1.25 C.)

Salt (to Taste)

Directions:

To begin this recipe, start by heating a pan over medium heat. Once warm, place the olive oil and maple in and bring to a boil.

Once boiling, stir in your hazelnuts and cook on high for a minute or two. After this time passes, add in the chia seeds and salt and cook for another three minutes.

Now, turn the heat down to low and begin crushing the hazelnuts in the pan before pouring onto a lined cookie sheet. At this point, try to spread the mixture evenly across the pan and then place it in the freezer for 15 minutes.

Once the mixture has completely cooled, chop the ingredients into clusters and enjoy.

Nutrition: Calories: 330 Proteins: 3g Carbs: 60g Fats: 11g

Honey Peanut Butter

Preparation time: 10 minutes

Cooking time: 0 minutes

Servings: 6

Ingredients

1 cup peanut butter

3/4 cup honey extracted

1/2 cup ground peanuts

1 tsp ground cinnamon

Directions:

Add all ingredients into your fast-speed blender, and blend until smooth.

Keep refrigerated.

Mediterranean Marinated Olives

Preparation time: 10 minutes

Cooking time: 0 minutes

Servings: 2

Ingredients

24 large olives, black, green, Kalamata

1/2 cup extra-virgin olive oil

4 cloves garlic, thinly sliced

2 Tbsp fresh lemon juice

2 tsp coriander seeds, crushed

1/2 tsp crushed red pepper

1 tsp dried thyme

1 tsp dried rosemary, crushed

Salt and ground pepper to taste

Directions:

Place olives and all remaining ingredients in a large container or bag, and shake to combine well.

Cover and refrigerate to marinate overnight.

Serve.

Keep refrigerated.

Nut Butter & Dates Granola

Preparation time: 1 hour

Cooking time: 55 minutes

Servings: 8

Ingredients

3 cups rolled oats

2 cups dates, pitted and chopped

1 cup flaked or shredded coconut

1/2 cup wheat germ

1/4 cup soy milk powder

1/2 cup almonds chopped

3/4 cup honey strained

1/2 cup almond butter (plain, unsalted) softened

1/4 cup peanut butter softened

Directions:

Preheat oven to 300F. Add all ingredients into a food processor and pulse until roughly combined. Spread mixture evenly into greased 10 x 15-inch baking pan. Bake for 45 to 55 minutes. Stir mixture several times during baking.

Remove from the oven and cool completely.

Store in a covered glass jar.

Oven-baked Caramelize Plantains

Preparation time: 30 minutes

Cooking time: 17 minutes

Servings: 4

Ingredients

4 medium plantains, peeled and sliced

2 Tbsp fresh orange juice

4 Tbsp brown sugar or to taste

1 Tbsp grated orange zest

4 Tbsp coconut butter, melted

Directions

Preheat oven to 360 F/180 C.

Place plantain slices in a heatproof dish.

Pour the orange juice over plantains, and then sprinkle with brown sugar and grated orange zest.

Melt coconut butter and pour evenly over plantains.

Cover with foil and bake for 15 to 17 minutes.

Serve warm or cold with honey or maple syrup.

Powerful Peas & Lentils Dip

Preparation time: 10 minutes

Cooking time: 0 minutes

Servings: 4

Ingredients

4 cups frozen peas

2 cup green lentils cooked

1 piece of grated ginger

1/2 cup fresh basil chopped

1 cup ground almonds

Juice of 1/2 lime

Pinch of salt

4 Tbsp sesame oil

1/4 cup Sesame seeds

Directions

Place all ingredients in a food processor or in a blender.

Blend until all ingredients combined well.

Keep refrigerated in an airtight container up to 4 days.

Avocado Hummus

Preparation time: 10 mins

Cooking time:

Servings: 4

Ingredients

2 Ripe Avocados

½ Cup Coconut Cream

¼ Cup Sesame Paste

½ Lemon Juice

1 Tsp. Clove, Pressed

½ Tsp Ground Cumin

½ Tsp Salt

¼ Tsp Ground Black Pepper

Directions

Cut the avocado lengthways and remove seed from the fruit.

Put all ingredients in a blender or food processor and mix until thoroughly smooth.

Add more cream, lemon juice or water if you want to have a looser texture.

Adjust seasonings as needed. Serve with naan and enjoy.

Nutrition: Protein: 6% 21 kcal Fat: 79% 289 kcal

Carbohydrates: 16% 57 kcal

Plant Based Crispy Falafel

Preparation time: 20 mins

Cooking time: 30 mins

Servings: 8

Ingredients

1 tbsp. extra-virgin olive oil

1 cup dried chickpeas soaked for 24 hours in the refrigerator

1 cup cauliflower, chopped

½ cup red onion, chopped

½ cup packed fresh parsley

2 cloves garlic, quartered

1 tsp. sea salt

½ tsp. ground black pepper

½ tsp. ground cumin

¼ tsp. ground cinnamon

Directions

Preheat oven to 375° F.

In a food processor, mix chickpeas, cauliflower, onion, parsley, garlic, salt, pepper, cumin seeds, cinnamon, and olive oil until mixture is smooth.

Take 2 tbsps. of mixture and make the falafel into small patties.

Keep falafel on greased baking tray.

Bake falafel for about 25 to 30 minutes in preheated oven until golden brown from both sides.

Once cooked remove from oven.

Serve hot fresh vegetable salad and enjoy!

Nutrition: Protein: 16% 19 kcal Fat: 24% 29 kcal Carbohydrates: 60% 71 kcal

Waffles With Almond Flour

Preparation time: 15 mins

Cooking time: 15 mins

Servings: 4

Ingredients

1 cup almond milk

2 tbsps. chia seeds

2 tsp lemon juice

4 tbsps. coconut oil

1/2 cup almond flour

2 tbsps. maple syrup

Cooking spray or cooking oil

Directions

Mix coconut milk with lemon juice in a mixing bowl.

Leave it for 5-8 minutes on room temperature to turn it into butter milk.

Once coconut milk is turned into butter milk, add chai seeds into milk and whisk together.

Add other ingredients in milk mixture and mix well.

Preheat a waffle iron and spray it with coconut oil spray.

Pour 2 tbsp. of waffle mixture into the waffle machine and cook until golden.

Top with some berries and serve hot.

Enjoy with black coffee!

Nutrition: Protein: 5% 15 kcal Fat: 71% 199 kcal Carbohydrates: 23% 66 kcal

Avocado And Tempeh Bacon Wraps

Preparation Time: 10 minutes

Cooking time: 8 minutes

Servings: 4 wraps

Ingredients

2 tablespoons olive oil

8 ounces tempeh bacon, homemade or store-bought

4 (10-inch) soft flour tortillas or lavash flatbread

1/4 cup vegan mayonnaise, homemade or store-bought

4 large lettuce leaves

2 ripe Hass avocados, pitted, peeled, and cut into 1/4-inch slices

1 large ripe tomato, cut into 1/4-inch slices

Directions

In a large skillet, heat the oil over medium heat. Add the tempeh bacon and cook until browned on both sides, about 8 minutes. Remove from the heat and set aside.

Place 1 tortilla on a work surface. Spread with some of the mayonnaise and one-fourth of the lettuce and tomatoes.

Pit, peel, and thinly slice the avocado and place the slices on top of the tomato. Add the reserved tempeh bacon and roll up tightly. Repeat with remaining Ingredients and serve.

Kale Chips

Preparation Time: 5 minutes Cooking time: 25 minutes

Servings: 2

Ingredients

1 large bunch kale

1 tablespoon extra-virgin olive oil

½ teaspoon chipotle powder

½ teaspoon smoked paprika

¼ teaspoon salt

Directions

Preparing the Ingredients.

Preheat the oven to 275°F.

Line a large baking sheet with parchment paper. In a large bowl, stem the kale and tear it into bite-size pieces. Add the olive oil, chipotle powder, smoked paprika, and salt.

Toss the kale with tongs or your hands, coating each piece well.

Spread the kale over the parchment paper in a single layer. Bake for 25 minutes, turning halfway through, until crisp. Cool for 10 to 15 minutes before dividing and storing in 2 airtight containers.

Nutrition: Calories: 144; Fat: 7g; Protein: 5g; Carbohydrates: 18g; Fiber: 3g; Sugar: 0g; Sodium: 363mg

Apple Cinnamon Crisps

Preparation Time: 2 Hours

Cooking Time: 2 Hours

Servings: 2

Ingredients:

Cinnamon (1 t.)

Apple (1, Sliced)

Directions:

This recipe is simple and delicious! You can start off by turning the oven to 200. As this warms up, you'll want to prep a baking sheet with some parchment paper.

With the baking sheet set, layout your apple slices across it evenly and sprinkle with the cinnamon. Once this is done, pop the dish into the oven for two hours.

Remove from oven, allow to cool, and enjoy.

Nutrition: Calories: 50 Proteins: 5g Carbs: 14g Fats: 1g

Flavour Boosters and Souce Recipes

Southwestern Oregano Thyme Rub

This rub is a perfect blend of herbal, sweet, and earthy ingredients to make your day truly special and delicious. If you wish to make your meat cuts less spicy, then you can adjust the quantity of chili powder.

Preparation Time: 5 min.

Cooking Time: 5 min.

Servings: 11 tbs.

Ingredients:

Garlic powder - 2 tbs.

Chili powder - 2 tbs.

Dry mustard - 2 tbs.

Dried thyme- 1 tbs.

Dried oregano - 1 tbs.

Mild paprika - 1 tbs.

Ground coriander - 1 tbs.

Ground cumin - 1 tbs.

Salt - 2 tsp.

Directions:

Mix all mentioned ingredients in your mixing bowl to make the oregano thyme rub. Gently mix all the ingredients using spatula or spoon to form an aromatic rub mixture.

Now, take your choice of meat cut and place it on a firm surface. Brush or rub the freshly made rub on it; pat gently for the rub to stick onto the surface. Turn the meat cut and repeat to spice up its other side. Repeat with other meat cuts.
The freshly rubbed meat is ready to be grilled or cooked!

Tangy Pepper & Thyme Rub

Transform your dry meats into full of citrusy, dark, and spicy flavors with this triple spice rub. The tangy thyme rub is quite easy to prepare and beautifully spices up your chicken, pork as well as beef.

Preparation Time: 5 min.

Cooking Time: 0 min.

Servings: 2 tbs.

Ingredients:

Dried thyme - 1tbs.

Lime zest, finely grated – 1 tbs.

Sea salt and black pepper as required

Directions:

Mix in all the ingredients in your mixing bowl to make the pepper and thyme rub. Gently mix all the ingredients using spatula or spoon to form an aromatic rub mixture.

Now, take your choice of meat cut and place it on a firm surface. Brush or rub the freshly made rub on it; pat gently for the rub to stick onto the surface. Turn the meat cut and repeat to spice up its other side. Repeat with other meat cuts.

The freshly rubbed meat is ready to be grilled or cooked!

Vegan Smokey Maple BBQ Sauce

Preparation time: 5 minutes

Cooking time: 5 minutes

Servings: 8

Ingredients:

1 tablespoon maple syrup

1/2 cup ketchup

1 teaspoon garlic powder

1 teaspoon liquid smoke

Directions:

Add all ingredients to a bowl. Mix them until well combined. Serve and enjoy.

Vegan Bean Pesto

Preparation time: 5 minutes

Cooking time: 5 minutes

Servings: 2

Ingredients

1 can (15 oz.) white beans, drained, rinsed

2 cups basil leaves, washed, dried

½ cup non-dairy milk

2 tablespoons olive oil

3 tablespoons nutritional yeast

1 garlic clove, peeled

Pepper and salt to taste

Directions:

Blend all the ingredients (except the seasonings) in a blender until smooth.

Sprinkle with pepper and salt to taste, then blend for 1 extra minute. Enjoy with pasta.

Meal Plans

Meal Plan 1

Day	Breakfast	Lunch	Dinner	Snacks
1	Chocolate PB Smoothie	Cauliflower Latke	Noodles Alfredo with Herby Tofu	Beans with Sesame Hummus
2	Orange french toast	Roasted Brussels Sprouts	Lemon Couscous with Tempeh Kabobs	Candied Honey-Coconut Peanuts
3	Oatmeal Raisin Breakfast Cookie	Brussels Sprouts & Cranberries Salad	Portobello Burger with Veggie Fries	Choco Walnuts Fat Bombs
4	Berry Beetsicle Smoothie	Potato Latke	Thai Seitan Vegetable Curry	Crispy Honey Pecans (Slow Cooker)
5	Blueberry Oat Muffins	Broccoli Rabe	Tofu Cabbage Stir-Fry	Crunchy Fried Pickles

6	Quinoa Applesauce Muffins	Whipped Potatoes	Curried Tofu with Buttery Cabbage	Granola bars with Maple Syrup
7	Pumpkin pancakes	Quinoa Avocado Salad	Smoked Tempeh with Broccoli Fritters	Green Soy Beans Hummus
8	Green breakfast smoothie	Roasted Sweet Potatoes	Cheesy Potato Casserole	High Protein Avocado Guacamole
9	Blueberry Lemonade Smoothie	Cauliflower Salad	Curry Mushroom Pie	Homemade Energy Nut Bars
10	Berry Protein Smoothie	Garlic Mashed Potatoes & Turnips	Spicy Cheesy Tofu Balls	Honey Peanut Butter
11	Blueberry and chia smoothie	Green Beans with Bacon	Radish Chips	Mediterranean Marinated Olives
12	Green Kickstart Smoothie	Coconut Brussels Sprouts	Sautéed Pears	Nut Butter & Dates Granola

13	Warm Maple and Cinnamon Quinoa	Cod Stew with Rice & Sweet Potatoes	Pecan & Blueberry Crumble	Oven-baked Caramelize Plantains
14	Warm Quinoa Breakfast Bowl	Chicken & Rice	Rice Pudding	Powerful Peas & Lentils Dip
15	Banana Bread Rice Pudding	Rice Bowl with Edamame	Mango Sticky Rice	Protein "Raffaello" Candies
16	Apple and cinnamon oatmeal	Chickpea Avocado Sandwich	Noodles Alfredo with Herby Tofu	Protein-Rich Pumpkin Bowl
17	Mango Key Lime Pie Smoothie	Roasted Tomato Sandwich	Lemon Couscous with Tempeh Kabobs	Savory Red Potato-Garlic Balls
18	Spiced orange breakfast couscous	Pulled "Pork" Sandwiches	Portobello Burger with Veggie Fries	Spicy Smooth Red Lentil Dip

19	Breakfast parfaits	Cauliflower Latke	Thai Seitan Vegetable Curry	Steamed Broccoli with Sesame
20	Sweet potato and kale hash	Roasted Brussels Sprouts	Tofu Cabbage Stir-Fry	Vegan Eggplant Patties
21	Delicious Oat Meal	Brussels Sprouts & Cranberries Salad	Curried Tofu with Buttery Cabbage	Vegan Breakfast Sandwich
22	Breakfast Cherry Delight	Potato Latke	Smoked Tempeh with Broccoli Fritters	Chickpea And Mushroom Burger
23	Crazy Maple and Pear Breakfast	Broccoli Rabe	Cheesy Potato Casserole	Beans with Sesame Hummus
24	Hearty French Toast Bowls	Whipped Potatoes	Curry Mushroom Pie	Candied Honey-Coconut Peanuts
25	Chocolate PB Smoothie	Quinoa Avocado Salad	Spicy Cheesy Tofu Balls	Choco Walnuts Fat Bombs

26	Orange french toast	Roasted Sweet Potatoes	Radish Chips	Crispy Honey Pecans (Slow Cooker)
27	Oatmeal Raisin Breakfast Cookie	Cauliflower Salad	Sautéed Pears	Crunchy Fried Pickles
28	Berry Beetsicle Smoothie	Garlic Mashed Potatoes & Turnips	Pecan & Blueberry Crumble	Granola bars with Maple Syrup

Meal Plan 2

Day	Breakfast	Lunch	Dinner	Smoothie
1	Mexican-Spiced Tofu Scramble	Teriyaki Tofu Stir-fry	Mushroom Steak	Chocolate Smoothie
2	Whole Grain Protein Bowl	Red Lentil and Quinoa Fritters	Spicy Grilled Tofu Steak	Chocolate Mint Smoothie
3	Healthy Breakfast Bowl	Green Pea Fritters	Piquillo Salsa Verde Steak	Cinnamon Roll Smoothie
4	Healthy Breakfast Bowl	Breaded Tofu Steaks	Butternut Squash Steak	Coconut Smoothie
5	Root Vegetable Hash With Avocado Crème	Chickpea and Edamame Salad	Cauliflower Steak Kicking Corn	Maca Almond Smoothie
6	Chocolate Strawberry Almond Protein Smoothie	Thai Tofu and Quinoa Bowls	Pistachio Watermelon Steak	Blueberry Smoothie
7	Banana Bread Breakfast Muffins	Black Bean and Bulgur Chili	BBQ Ribs	Nutty Protein Shake

8	Stracciatella Muffins	Cauliflower Steaks	Spicy Veggie Steaks With veggies	Cinnamon Pear Smoothie
9	Cardamom Persimmon Scones With Maple-Persimmon Cream	Avocado and Hummus Sandwich	Mushroom Steak	Vanilla Milkshake
10	Activated Buckwheat & Coconut Porridge With Blueberry Sauce	Chickpea Spinach Salad	Spicy Grilled Tofu Steak	Raspberry Protein Shake
11	Sweet Molasses Brown Bread	Teriyaki Tofu Stir-fry	Piquillo Salsa Verde Steak	Raspberry Almond Smoothie
12	Mexican-Spiced Tofu Scramble	Red Lentil and Quinoa Fritters	Butternut Squash Steak	Chocolate Smoothie
13	Whole Grain Protein Bowl	Green Pea Fritters	Cauliflower Steak Kicking Corn	Chocolate Mint Smoothie
14	Healthy Breakfast Bowl	Breaded Tofu Steaks	Pistachio Watermelon Steak	Cinnamon Roll Smoothie

15	Healthy Breakfast Bowl	Chickpea and Edamame Salad	BBQ Ribs	Coconut Smoothie
16	Root Vegetable Hash With Avocado Crème	Thai Tofu and Quinoa Bowls	Spicy Veggie Steaks With veggies	Maca Almond Smoothie
17	Chocolate Strawberry Almond Protein Smoothie	Black Bean and Bulgur Chili	Mushroom Steak	Blueberry Smoothie
18	Banana Bread Breakfast Muffins	Cauliflower Steaks	Spicy Grilled Tofu Steak	Nutty Protein Shake
19	Stracciatella Muffins	Avocado and Hummus Sandwich	Piquillo Salsa Verde Steak	Cinnamon Pear Smoothie
20	Cardamom Persimmon Scones With Maple-Persimmon Cream	Chickpea Spinach Salad	Butternut Squash Steak	Vanilla Milkshake

21	Activated Buckwheat & Coconut Porridge With Blueberry Sauce	Teriyaki Tofu Stir-fry	Cauliflower Steak Kicking Corn	Raspberry Protein Shake
22	Sweet Molasses Brown Bread	Red Lentil and Quinoa Fritters	Pistachio Watermelon Steak	Raspberry Almond Smoothie
23	Mexican-Spiced Tofu Scramble	Green Pea Fritters	BBQ Ribs	Chocolate Smoothie
24	Whole Grain Protein Bowl	Breaded Tofu Steaks	Spicy Veggie Steaks With veggies	Chocolate Mint Smoothie
25	Healthy Breakfast Bowl	Chickpea and Edamame Salad	Mushroom Steak	Cinnamon Roll Smoothie
26	Healthy Breakfast Bowl	Thai Tofu and Quinoa Bowls	Spicy Grilled Tofu Steak	Coconut Smoothie
27	Root Vegetable Hash With Avocado Crème	Black Bean and Bulgur Chili	Piquillo Salsa Verde Steak	Maca Almond Smoothie

| 28 | Chocolate Strawberry Almond Protein Smoothie | Cauliflower Steaks | Butternut Squash Steak | Blueberry Smoothie |

Meal Plan 3

Day	Breakfast	Lunch	Dinner	Snacks
1	Breakfast Blueberry Muffins	Quinoa Buddha Bowl	Broccoli & black beans stir fry	Spiced Chickpeas
2	Oatmeal with Pears	Lettuce Hummus Wrap	Stuffed peppers	Lemon & Ginger Kale Chips
3	Yogurt with Cucumber	Simple Curried Vegetable Rice	Sweet 'n spicy tofu	Chocolate Energy Snack Bar
4	Breakfast Casserole	Spicy Southwestern Hummus Wraps	Eggplant & mushrooms in peanut sauce	Hazelnut & Maple Chia Crunch
5	Berries with Mascarpone on Toasted Bread	Buffalo Cauliflower Wings	Green beans stir fry	Roasted Cauliflower
6	Fruit Cup	Veggie Fritters	Collard greens 'n tofu	Apple Cinnamon Crisps
7	Oatmeal with Black Beans & Cheddar	Pizza Bites	Cassoulet	Pumpkin Spice Granola Bites

8	Breakfast Smoothie	Avocado, Spinach and Kale Soup	Double-garlic bean and vegetable soup	Salted Carrot Fries
9	Yogurt with Beets & Raspberries	Curry spinach soup	Mean bean minestrone	Zesty Orange Muffins
10	Curry Oatmeal	Arugula and Artichokes Bowls	Grilled Halloumi Broccoli Salad	Chocolate Tahini Balls
11	Fig & Cheese Oatmeal	Minty arugula soup	Black Bean Lentil Salad With Lime Dressing	Spiced Chickpeas
12	Pumpkin Oats	Spinach and Broccoli Soup	Arugula Lentil Salad	Lemon & Ginger Kale Chips
13	Sweet Potato Toasts	Coconut zucchini cream	Red Cabbage Salad With Curried Seitan	Chocolate Energy Snack Bar
14	Tofu Scramble Tacos	Zucchini and Cauliflower Soup	Chickpea, Red Kidney Bean And Feta Salad	Hazelnut & Maple Chia Crunch

15	Almond Chia Pudding	Chard soup	The Amazing Chickpea Spinach Salad	Roasted Cauliflower
16	Breakfast Parfait Popsicles	Avocado, Pine Nuts and Chard Salad	Curried Carrot Slaw With Tempeh	Apple Cinnamon Crisps
17	Strawberry Smoothie Bowl	Grapes, Avocado and Spinach Salad	Black & White Bean Quinoa Salad	Pumpkin Spice Granola Bites
18	Peanut Butter Granola	Greens and Olives Pan	Greek Salad With Seitan Gyros Strips	Salted Carrot Fries
19	Apple Chia Pudding	Mushrooms and Chard Soup	Chickpea And Edamame Salad	Zesty Orange Muffins
20	Pumpkin Spice Bites	Tomato, Green Beans and Chard Soup	Broccoli & black beans stir fry	Chocolate Tahini Balls
21	Lemon Spelt Scones	Hot roasted peppers cream	Stuffed peppers	Spiced Chickpeas
22	Veggie Breakfast Scramble	Eggplant and Peppers Soup	Sweet 'n spicy tofu	Lemon & Ginger Kale Chips

23	Breakfast Blueberry Muffins	Eggplant and Olives Stew	Eggplant & mushrooms in peanut sauce	Chocolate Energy Snack Bar
24	Oatmeal with Pears	Cauliflower and Artichokes Soup	Green beans stir fry	Hazelnut & Maple Chia Crunch
25	Yogurt with Cucumber	Quinoa Buddha Bowl	Collard greens 'n tofu	Roasted Cauliflower
26	Breakfast Casserole	Lettuce Hummus Wrap	Cassoulet	Apple Cinnamon Crisps
27	Berries with Mascarpone on Toasted Bread	Simple Curried Vegetable Rice	Double-garlic bean and vegetable soup	Pumpkin Spice Granola Bites
28	Fruit Cup	Spicy Southwestern Hummus Wraps	Mean bean minestrone	Salted Carrot Fries

Meal plan 4

Day	Breakfast	Entrées	Soup, Salad, & Sides	Smoothie
1	Tasty Oatmeal Muffins	Black Bean Dip	Spinach Soup with Dill and Basil	Fruity Smoothie
2	Omelet with Chickpea Flour	Cannellini Bean Cashew Dip	Coconut Watercress Soup	Energizing Ginger Detox Tonic
3	White Sandwich Bread	Cauliflower Popcorn	Coconut Watercress Soup	Warm Spiced Lemon Drink
4	A Toast to Remember	Cinnamon Apple Chips with Dip	Coconut Watercress Soup	Soothing Ginger Tea Drink
5	Tasty Panini	Crunchy Asparagus Spears	Cauliflower Spinach Soup	Nice Spiced Cherry Cider

6	Tasty Oatmeal and Carrot Cake	Cucumber Bites with Chive and Sunflower Seeds	Avocado Mint Soup	Fragrant Spiced Coffee
7	Onion & Mushroom Tart with a Nice Brown Rice Crust	Garlicky Kale Chips	Creamy Squash Soup	Tangy Spiced Cranberry Drink
8	Perfect Breakfast Shake	Hummus-stuffed Baby Potatoes	Cucumber Edamame Salad	Warm Pomegranate Punch
9	Beet Gazpacho	Homemade Trail Mix	Best Broccoli Salad	Rich Truffle Hot Chocolate
10	Vegetable Rice	Nut Butter Maple Dip	Rainbow Orzo Salad	Ultimate Mulled Wine
11	Courgette Risotto	Oven Baked Sesame Fries	Broccoli Pasta Salad	Pleasant Lemonade
12	Country Breakfast Cereal	Pumpkin Orange Spice Hummus	Eggplant & Roasted Tomato Farro Salad	Pineapple, Banana & Spinach Smoothie

13	Oatmeal Fruit Shake	Quick English Muffin Mexican Pizzas	Garden Patch Sandwiches on Multigrain Bread	Kale & Avocado Smoothie
14	Amaranth Banana Breakfast Porridge	Quinoa Trail Mix Cups	Garden Salad Wraps	Coconut & Strawberry Smoothie
15	Green Ginger Smoothie	Black Bean Dip	Marinated Mushroom Wraps	Pumpkin Chia Smoothie
16	Orange Dream Creamsicle	Cannellini Bean Cashew Dip	Tamari Toasted Almonds	Cantaloupe Smoothie Bowl
17	Strawberry Limeade	Cauliflower Popcorn	Nourishing Whole-Grain Porridge	Berry & Cauliflower Smoothie
18	Peanut Butter and Jelly Smoothie	Cinnamon Apple Chips with Dip	Pungent Mushroom Barley Risotto	Green Mango Smoothie

19	Banana Almond Granola	Crunchy Asparagus Spears	Spinach Soup with Dill and Basil	Chia Seed Smoothie
20	Tasty Oatmeal Muffins	Cucumber Bites with Chive and Sunflower Seeds	Coconut Watercress Soup	Mango Smoothie
21	Omelet with Chickpea Flour	Garlicky Kale Chips	Coconut Watercress Soup	Fruity Smoothie

CPSIA information can be obtained
at www.ICGtesting.com
Printed in the USA
LVHW080555120521
687119LV00007B/191